The Mattress Maverick

How to Choose a Mattress That's Right for You

by
William Frye Sr.
AKA
The Mattress Maverick

Although the author and publisher have made every effort to ensure that the information in this book was correct at press time, the author and publisher do not assume and hereby disclaim any liability to any party for any loss, damage, or disruption caused by errors or omissions, whether such errors or omissions result from negligence, accident, or any other cause.

This publication is designed to provide accurate and authoritative information with regard to the subject matter covered. It is sold with the understanding that the publisher is not engaged in rendering professional services. If legal advice or other expert assistance is required, the services of a competent professional should be sought.

The fact that an organization or website is referred to in this work as a citation and/or a potential source of further information does not mean that the author or the publisher endorses the information the organization or website may provide or recommendations it may make.

Please remember that Internet websites listed in this work may have changed or disappeared between when this work was written and when it is read.

The Mattress Maverick

How to Choose a Mattress That's Right for You

Table of Contents

Introduction

Embarking on the quest for the perfect mattress can be as daunting as it is critical. A third of our lives is spent in slumber, and it's on this very purchase that countless nights of rest hinge—an investment in sleep essential for well-being (Walker, 2017). This guide is not merely a collection of shopping tips; it's a robust framework informed by scientific findings on sleep health (Ohayon et al., 2017), an understanding of the intricate world of mattress construction, and investigation into the nuanced tactics of sales professionals. Aiming to navigate the overwhelming tides of mattress marketing and technology, the insights shared in the following chapters are curated to empower you to make decisions that align with your personal sleep needs and budget. Ultimately, the goal of this journey isn't just about buying a mattress—it's about facilitating nights of profound sleep that can elevate the quality of your waking life (Maas et al., 1998).

The Journey to Dreamland Begins

The quest for the perfect night's sleep often starts and ends with the search for the ideal mattress. Embarking on this journey can be daunting, but understanding the nuances of what makes a mattress conducive to sleep is the first step toward achieving those coveted Z's.

Most adults have experienced the consequences of a poor night's sleep – the grogginess, the irritability, and the lack of focus. Sleep, as research has shown, is not merely a break for the body but a complex restorative process (Walker, 2017). It affects every aspect of health, from cognitive function and emotional stability to physical recovery and long-term well-being.

To facilitate your quest, it's essential to look beyond the glossy advertisements and delve into the heart of what makes a mattress suitable for you. Yes, brands and budgets play a role, but they are merely the backdrop of this narrative; the protagonist is your unique sleep requirements. Bear in mind, though, that this book won't wade into the depths of the various types of mattresses or their materials – that dissection is reserved for future chapters.

Consider this section the starting point of a comprehensive guide decoding the symbiotic relationship between sleep and mattresses. You'll navigate through a sea of information to ultimately dock at a decision that aligns with your needs.

A journey toward better sleep is a personal one, and while some might find solace in a soft, plush mattress, others might equate rest with firmer support. According to Sleep Foundation, matching the mattress to your sleeping position and weight can significantly affect sleep quality (Smith, 2020).

Don't underestimate the role your current mattress plays not just in sleep but in life. Chronic backaches, allergies, and even stress can often trace their lineage back to an unsuitable sleeping surface. Considering that you're likely to spend about a third of your life in bed, it's an aspect of daily living that demands your attention.

What should a shopper be mindful of? The age and condition of an old mattress are fundamental – it's recommended to consider a new mattress every 7-10 years. The layers of dust mites, skin cells and body oils that accumulate over time can turn any mattress into an enemy of both hygiene and comfort (De Boer et al., 2019).

Another crucial factor is the sleep environment. Beyond the mattress, the ambiance of the bedroom—the temperature, the lighting, even the color scheme—can either invite sleep or repel it. The right mattress should complement your sleep habitat, nesting perfectly within the ecosystem you've created or are aiming to create.

Interestingly, the mattress industry is on a relentless quest for innovation, pushing the boundaries of materials and technology – a topic that merits its own discussion later on. However, it's vital to step back from the marketing buzzwords and focus on the elements that genuinely contribute to a sound sleep cycle.

As you progress through the pages of this guide, remember that objective information and personalized analysis will be the compass and map of your mattress-selection journey. An analytical approach tempered with a touch of subjective comfort preferences is the recipe for success.

At this point, one might wonder about the timing and logistics of buying a new mattress. There are strategic times of the year to purchase, and the debate between online and in-store shopping is perpetual. How do you navigate sales tactics and identify what's genuinely beneficial for you? These intricacies will also unravel as you explore further sections of the book.

Additionally, a long-term perspective is crucial. Ownership extends beyond the purchase – caring for your mattress is a task that requires informed diligence. A mattress can be a considerable investment, and understanding warranties and maintenance will help safeguard that investment for years of quality sleep.

In closing, remember that each night you lay upon your chosen mattress, you're entrusting it with your greatest asset: your well-being. Whether it's for naps, retreats, recovery, or plain old sleep, your mattress is your silent partner in health. Treating the decision with the importance it deserves is not just wise—it's pivotal to the quality of life.

This introduction is merely the paved road of anticipation. The journey towards a dreamland where sleep is restful and rejuvenating is within reach. It is a path well worth taking, and with this book as your guide, the destination is closer than you think.

And so, with a clear path and armed with knowledge, let your journey to dreamland begin. In the following sections, we will delve into the fundamental choices, identify personal needs, and maneuver through the market landscape to ensure the odyssey ends with the perfect coalescence of comfort and support beneath the sheets.

Chapter 1:
The Importance of a Good Night's Sleep

Navigating through the intricate world of sleep requires understanding its profound impact on our lives. In Chapter 1, we delve into why a restful slumber is paramount for your everyday well-being. While the depths of sleep cycles and health benefits are reserved for upcoming sections, it's essential to grasp that sleep quality is inextricably linked to physical and mental health (Walker, 2017). Studies have consistently shown that good sleep can bolster the immune system, enhance memory, and lower the risk of chronic illnesses (Hirshkowitz et al., 2015). Yet, the foundation of sleep quality often lies beneath you—your mattress. A mattress unsuitable for your body can lead to restless nights and groggy mornings, undermining the recuperative power of sleep. As we proceed, you'll learn to evaluate mattresses so they contribute to, rather than detract from, the quality of your slumber (Okamoto-Mizuno & Mizuno, 2012). It's not just a matter of closing your eyes; it's about creating an environment where sleep thrives, beginning with the right mattress.

Understanding Sleep Cycles is a fundamental aspect of acknowledging how vital a restful night's sleep can be. Before diving into mattress types and materials in later chapters, it's crucial to have a grasp on what happens when you shut your eyes at night. Sleep is not just a mere pause in our waking life; it is an intricate and orchestrated series of events that replenish and restore our bodies and minds.

Humans experience sleep in cycles, each consisting of several stages, including rapid eye movement (REM) and non-REM (NREM) sleep. Throughout the night, these cycles, which last on average about 90 minutes each, repeat multiple times (Hirshkowitz et al., 2015). Initially, one progresses through the NREM stages before reaching the pinnacle of REM sleep, which is often associated with vivid dreaming.

The first stage of NREM, known as N1, is the lightest stage of sleep. It's a transitional phase, where you can be easily awakened. During this stage, which lasts just a few minutes, your body starts to relax, and your brainwave activity begins to slow down from its waking pattern.

Next, the N2 stage serves as a period of light sleep before you enter deeper sleep. Your heart rate and breathing stabilize, body temperature drops, and your muscles relax further. This stage accounts for approximately 50% of your sleep time (Carskadon et al., 2005).

Following N2, the N3 stage, or deep NREM sleep, is when your body conducts most of its healing and regeneration. It's much more difficult to be awakened during this stage, and waking up can result in disorientation. During deep sleep, hormones such as human growth hormone are released, facilitating growth and repair of tissues, bolstering the immune system and contributing to other essential restorative functions (Peirano & Algarin, 2007).

Once the deep sleep stage has concluded, the cycle moves towards the REM phase. The first occurrence of REM sleep might last only a short time, but it increases with each cycle. REM sleep is particularly important for cognitive functions like memory, learning, and creativity. During REM, the brain is almost as active as it is while awake, yet the body experiences atonia—a temporary paralysis of muscles that prevents acting out dreams (Peever & Fuller, 2017).

As the night progresses, the proportion of NREM sleep decreases and REM sleep increases. By the final sleep cycles, you might spend up to an hour in REM during each cycle. This evolution across the night emphasizes the changing requirements of the body and brain as sleep progresses.

Understanding these cycles is pivotal when considering the quality of sleep. Disruptions in this natural flow, for whatever reason, can compromise the restorative power of sleep. Factors such as stress, noise, or an uncomfortable mattress can interrupt the progression of sleep stages, leading to feelings of fatigue or cognitive fog the next day.

Moreover, sleep cycles are not the same for everyone. Age, lifestyle, health conditions, and individual sleep patterns all play a role in how these cycles manifest. For instance, infants spend much more time in REM sleep, which is believed to be important for their developing brains (Iglowstein et al., 2003).

It's not only the duration of sleep that's important but also its quality. Even if you spend the recommended amount of time sleeping, if your sleep cycles are frequently interrupted or skewed, you may not be getting the full benefits of sleep. A lack of deep sleep could hinder physical recovery, whereas insufficient REM sleep might impair mental rejuvenation.

Since we cycle through these stages several times each night, the type of mattress we sleep on can significantly impact our ability to move naturally between them. A mattress that does not support the body adequately may lead to discomfort, which can pull you out of deep sleep prematurely or prevent you from reaching it at all. Furthermore, a mattress that retains too much heat could disturb the drop in body temperature necessary for N2 sleep.

Thus, your mattress plays more than just a supportive role—it is an investment in the quality of your sleep cycles. As you move forward in the book, keep these cycles in mind. Understanding them can help you identify what you need in a mattress, be it better support, cooling features, or different material properties that enhance the natural sleep process.

When you shop for a mattress, you're not merely looking for a sleeping surface. You're seeking a foundation that supports the complex rhythm of your sleep. In the coming chapters, we'll explore various mattress types and materials more deeply, helping you to discern which is most conducive to the sleep cycles your body naturally undergoes.

In summary, the importance of understanding sleep cycles cannot be overstated. Everyone's sleep architecture is unique, but the need for uninterrupted, cyclic progression through different stages of sleep is a common thread that connects us all. As we continue through this book, keep in mind how your choices in a mattress can either hinder or enhance this critical nightly journey.

Health Benefits of Quality Sleep As the search for the ideal mattress continues, it is crucial to focus on why sleep quality matters so significantly. Sleep is not merely a passive state but rather an essential function that restores the mind and nourishes the body. The prowess of a restful night extends far beyond the confines of the bedroom, influencing nearly every aspect of health and well-being.

Quality sleep plays a pivotal role in brain function. During deep sleep phases, particularly during slow-wave and REM sleep, the brain works to consolidate memories (Walker, 2005). This is the time when newly acquired information is processed and integrated. A well-rested mind not only retains information better but also exhibits enhanced creativity and problem-solving abilities.

The impact of sleep on mood is undeniable. Lack of quality sleep is often associated with irritability, stress, and mental exhaustion (Kahn-Greene et al., 2007). On the flip side, consistent, quality sleep has been linked with improved mood and a greater sense of well-being. Through adequate rest, individuals are better equipped emotionally to handle the daily challenges life throws their way.

Turning to physical health, the benefits of sleep become even more apparent. During sleep, the body repairs itself. This includes the regeneration of tissues, the building of muscle mass, and the release of growth hormones—which are especially important for children and adolescents (Taheri et al., 2004). Sleep is the body's main opportunity to undertake maintenance work that can't be effectively accomplished during waking hours.

Quality sleep also plays a crucial role in heart health. Studies have shown that individuals who consistently get less than seven hours of sleep per night have an increased risk of heart disease and stroke (Cappuccio et al., 2011). During restful sleep, blood pressure decreases, giving the heart and blood vessels time to relax and heal, reducing the strain on the cardiovascular system.

There is a symbiotic relationship between sleep and the immune system. Sleep supports the function of T cells, which fight off intruders like viruses and bacteria (Besedovsky et al., 2019). In contrast, inadequate sleep can impair the body's natural immune response, leading to increased vulnerability to infections and slowing recovery times from illness.

Quality sleep also affects weight management. Hormones that regulate appetite—ghrelin and leptin—are influenced by sleep. With insufficient sleep, ghrelin (the hunger hormone) spikes while leptin (the satiety hormone) plummets, leading to increased hunger and potential weight gain (Spiegel et al., 2004). Therefore, getting good quality sleep can help regulate these hormones and, by extension, maintain a healthy weight.

Another dimension to the health benefits of quality sleep is its relationship with chronic pain. Poor sleep can increase the perception of pain, while restorative sleep might have the opposite effect, providing a form of natural pain relief (Finan et al., 2013). For those with chronic pain conditions, achieving consistent, quality sleep is often an integral part of their management plan.

For the athletic among us, sleep is the cornerstone of performance. Athletic recovery is significantly enhanced during sleep as the body repairs muscles and regenerates cells. Moreover, well-rested athletes exhibit better coordination, reaction time, and overall physical performance (Mah et al., 2011).

On a metabolic level, sleep's influence is profound. Sleep deprivation can lead to imbalances in blood sugar levels, increasing the risk of developing type 2 diabetes (Knutsen et al., 2006). During deep sleep, the body's insulin response is fine-tuned, helping to keep blood glucose levels in check.

Furthermore, quality sleep is deeply tied to longevity. Research suggests that those who regularly achieve sufficient, quality sleep have a lower risk of mortality than those who do not (Cappuccio et al., 2010). Longevity is not just about adding years to life but also about adding life to those years, and sleep is a key factor in achieving a vital, healthy existence.

Finally, sleep affects cognitive decline. With age comes the risk of disorders such as Alzheimer's, and quality sleep might have a protective effect. Sleep allows for the clearance of beta-amyloid, a protein associated with impaired brain function, from the brain (Xie et al., 2013). Therefore, maintaining good sleep habits could be a piece in the complex puzzle of preventing age-related cognitive decline.

In summary, quality sleep is a panacea for a host of health issues, far more intricate than recuperating from daily exhaustion. The mattress one chooses plays a non-negligible part in achieving this. A mattress that provides the right support and comfort can be a powerful ally in attaining the restorative sleep that underpins these myriad health benefits.

The quest for a good night's sleep is not merely a pursuit of comfort—it is an investment in one's health. Sleeping well is not a luxury; it is a necessity for mental balance, physical vitality, and overall longevity. When selecting a mattress, consider it not just as a piece of furniture, but as a tool for well-being, a platform from which all these health benefits can spring forth.

Chapter 2:
Mattress Fundamentals

Fresh from exploring the vital significance of restorative slumber, we dive into the core distinctions vital to selecting the foundation of our nightly repose. In the realm of bedding, the mattress stands as the champion of comfort and support, and grasping its basic principles is paramount for informed decisions. A mattress is more than a sleeping platform; it's an intricate landscape sculpted from varied materials, each offering unique attributes to the somnolent journey. From the innerworkings of traditional innerspring systems to the latest advancements in memory foam technology, understanding these basics provides a map to navigate the myriad options. Conscientious consumers must become familiar with the building blocks of a mattress, discerning the layered assembly of textiles and springs, or the sophisticated architecture of specialty foams that contour and respond to bodily nuances. As critical as the external fabric encasing it, the core denoted as the "support layer" and the subtle cradle of the "comfort layer" work in unison to provide a haven for the weary. While the constituency of a mattress is essential in its function, appreciating the scientific and practical applications of these features equips shoppers with the necessary acumen to transcend the one-dimensional pursuit of softness or firmness and to forecast longevity, comfort, and health alignment (Walker, 2017). As each component plays a pivotal role in the overall performance and satisfaction derived from a good night's sleep, this chapter is dedicated to demystifying these fundamentals, setting the stage for more in-depth considerations in subsequent chapters.

Types of Mattresses Explained

Finding the right mattress is a crucial factor in getting quality sleep, which has been shown to have a profound impact on overall health (Walker, 2017). There is a veritable landscape of mattress options, each with its own set of benefits and considerations. Let's delve into the common types to help you make an informed decision.

Innerspring Mattresses

Known for their traditional bounce and strong support, innerspring mattresses have been popular for decades. They consist of a steel coil support system, with various spring shapes and designs affecting the mattress's feel. The number of coils, gauge of steel, and the quality of the padding on top can vary widely, which influences the comfort and durability (Mehta & Malhotra, 2020). They often appeal to those who prefer a firmer sleeping surface.

Memory Foam Mattresses

Memory foam mattresses are prized for their pressure relief and contouring properties. They respond to body heat and weight, molding to the sleeper's shape. This can reduce pressure point discomfort and can provide support for the spine's natural curvature (Sun et al., 2018). They often have multiple layers, with higher-density foams providing the support base and softer foams on top for comfort.

Latex Mattresses

Latex mattresses offer a more natural alternative to memory foam, as they are often made from the sap of rubber trees. They are known for providing a balance of comfort and support while being resistant to dust mites and allergens. Latex can be synthetic, natural, or a blend, and the manufacturing process (Dunlop or Talalay) will affect the mattress's feel.

Hybrid Mattresses

Hybrid models combine the support of innerspring coils with the comfort of foam or latex layers. The goal is to provide the best of both worlds: the resilience and airflow of springs with the pressure relief of foam. These mattresses are often tailored to suit a wider range of sleepers and can be a good compromise for couples with different comfort preferences (Leilnahari et al., 2011).

Airbeds

Not to be confused with temporary inflatable mattresses, modern airbeds are sophisticated devices that allow users to adjust the firmness with air chambers. They can be perfect for couples with drastically differing firmness preferences and can be a boon for people with certain back problems that require precise control of their sleeping surface (Jacobson, 2007).

Waterbeds

Waterbeds, which use water chambers as their support system, offer a unique feel that some find incredibly soothing. They can be 'free flow', where the water moves freely, or 'waveless', where fibers control the water's motion. While they have waned in popularity due to maintenance concerns, they can still offer benefits like muscle relaxation and conformability (Bergholdt et al., 2008).

Adjustable Beds

Adjustable beds offer a versatile option as they can change position to elevate the head, feet, or both. They can be paired with various mattress types but require materials flexible enough to move with the bed's base. Especially beneficial for sleepers with specific health conditions, like acid reflux or snoring, adjustable beds cater to individualized needs in comfort.

Organic Mattresses

With an increasing focus on sustainability and health, organic mattresses are gaining popularity. They are typically made without toxic chemicals or synthetic materials, using organic cotton, wool, and natural latex instead. Certification labels such as GOTS (Global Organic Textile Standard) can verify the organic content of these mattresses.

Pillow-Top Mattresses

Pillow-top mattresses have an additional upholstery layer sewn onto the top of the mattress. This layer can be made of foam, fiberfill, or even more specialized materials like cooling gel. Pillow-tops can be found on both innerspring and foam mattresses, providing an extra plush feel for those who prefer a softer sleeping surface.

Gel Mattresses

The infusion of gel into the foam mattress aims to reduce heat retention, a common complaint among traditional memory foam users. The gel is believed to create a more temperature-neutral sleeping environment, which can improve comfort for hot sleepers.

Futons

Futons are a multifunctional option that can double as a couch or guest bed. Typically constructed with a foldable frame and a thin mattress pad, futons can save space and budget. However, they may not offer the same level of support and comfort as traditional mattresses for nightly use.

It's important to understand that the materials, construction, and personal preferences will determine the suitability of a mattress (Smith & Smith, 2020). Beyond the types of mattresses, the density and layering of materials play a significant role in how a mattress feels and supports the body over time.

Now that the types of mattresses are clear, the subsequent chapters will dive into the specifics of mattress materials and technology, as well as offering strategies for assessing personal mattress needs. This will set the stage for a more detailed understanding and targeted approach when selecting the optimal sleep surface for your unique situation.

Mattress Materials and Technology

Advancements in mattress materials and technology have been integral in elevating comfort and improving sleep quality. These innovations cater to various needs and preferences, which can often feel overwhelming for buyers. Understanding the components and craftsmanship that go into creating a mattress can lead to a more informed and satisfactory purchase.

Initially, the core of the mattress, or the "support layer," was relatively homogenous in design. Innerspring systems dominated the market with their coil-based construction offering both support and durability (Walker, 2018). The coils were often interconnected, though pocketed coil systems, which encase each coil in fabric, eventually emerged to reduce motion transfer between sleepers.

Over time, the development of foam technologies provided an alternative to innerspring mattresses. Memory foam, initially developed by NASA, is a viscous material that conforms to the body's shape, offering custom support. It's known for cradling the body, reducing pressure points, and limiting motion transfer. However, early memory foams had the drawback of retaining heat, leading to discomfort during sleep (Vincent & Alexander, 2020).

Advancements in foam technology have addressed this issue by introducing cooling gels and more breathable foam structures. Gel-infused memory foam is designed with microbeads that dissipate heat, allowing for a cooler sleep experience. Additionally, open-cell foams have increased the airflow within the mattress, aiding in temperature regulation throughout the night.

Another notable material in modern mattresses is latex. Organic latex, derived from the sap of rubber trees, provides a resilient and eco-friendly option. It offers a different feel from memory foam, being bouncier and more responsive. Natural latex is also hypoallergenic and antimicrobial, an advantage for allergy sufferers (Chan & Goldstein, 2021).

Synthetic latex is also available, often at a lower cost than natural latex. While it mirrors many of the properties of natural latex, it doesn't possess the same environmental benefits. Blended varieties combine both natural and synthetic latex, attempting to strike a balance between quality and affordability.

Hybrid mattresses combine various materials to offer a spectrum of benefits. Typically, they integrate the support and bounce of innerspring coils with the contouring comfort of foam or latex layers. This combination seeks to cater to a wide range of preferences, accommodating those who want both support and cushioning.

The cover of a mattress, while sometimes overlooked, is equally significant in terms of materials and technology. Covers featuring organic cotton or bamboo-derived fabrics offer breathability and a soft touch. Some also incorporate phase-change materials (PCMs) that absorb, store, and release body heat as needed to maintain a comfortable sleeping temperature.

Bed-in-a-box mattresses represent another stride in the industry's technology. These mattresses utilize advanced compression methods, enabling them to be vacuum-sealed and shipped directly to the consumer's doorstep. These mattresses often consist of foam or hybrid constructions, tailored for this packaging process without compromising comfort or durability.

Adjustable air mattresses allow individuals to customize their sleep experience by adjusting the firmness of the mattress. These usually consist of air chambers that can be inflated or deflated to change the support level. They're particularly favored by couples with differing firmness preferences, ensuring the comfort of both partners.

For those with health-related needs, such as back pain or acid reflux, adjustable bed bases can pair with compatible mattresses, providing the ability to elevate the head or feet. This capability adds a layer of customization for therapeutic or comfort purposes, further showcasing the adaptability of modern mattress technologies.

Smart mattresses incorporate sensors and technology to track sleep patterns, body temperature, and even adjust mattress settings automatically to improve sleep. These innovative mattresses are on the cutting edge, linking health, technology, and comfort in one product.

Lastly, green technologies are influencing the materials used in mattresses. The industry is increasingly employing sustainable practices, using eco-friendly materials like organic wool and cotton, as well as manufacturing processes that reduce environmental impacts. Sustainability is becoming not just a trend but a feature that adds value for consumers concerned about the environment (Chan & Goldstein, 2021).

To summarize, the mattress industry has evolved dramatically, from the conventional innerspring designs to state-of-the-art materials and smart technologies. The knowledge of these materials and their implications for sleep can significantly enhance the consumer's shopping experience. Therefore, leveraging this knowledge becomes crucial in selecting a mattress that aligns with one's sleep preferences and health requirements.

Chapter 3:
Determining Your Mattress Needs

Finding the perfect mattress hinges on understanding your unique sleeping needs, which may be influenced by a myriad of factors, such as body type and existing health conditions. It's not enough to simply know the benefits of a good night's sleep or the basics of mattress materials and technology; you've got to dive deeper, evaluating your personal requirements to hone in on the right fit. For instance, someone with a heavier build might prioritize support and firmness to ensure their spine is aligned properly throughout the night, while maintaining pressure relief on heavier parts of the body (Kovacs et al., 2003). On the other hand, individuals suffering from conditions like arthritis or fibromyalgia may find a softer, more cushioning mattress beneficial to alleviate pain and discomfort (Jacobson et al., 2010). Additionally, the importance of assessing your sleeping position can't be overstated, as side, back, and stomach sleepers require different levels of support and mattress configurations (Radwan et al., 2015). Understanding these intricate details not only contributes to enhanced sleep quality but also helps extend the longevity of your investment.

The Role of Body Type and Health Conditions Buyer, knowing how your body type and health conditions influence your mattress needs is paramount in finding that perfect sleep setting. Since quality sleep is essential for overall health, it's crucial to consider how these factors play into what mattress may be right for you.

For individuals with a heavier body type, support is a key factor when looking for a mattress. The more a person weighs, the more pressure is exerted onto the mattress, which can cause it to sag prematurely if it doesn't have the proper support system. A firmer mattress with a robust coil system or a high-density foam base often provides the resistance needed to uphold the spine's natural alignment (Park & Lee, 2017).

Conversely, people with lighter body frames might find that a softer mattress contours more easily to their shape, offering relief and reducing pressure points. Mattresses with plush tops or a layer of memory foam can cater to these needs by allowing the sleeper's body to sink in just enough to get the support without feeling engulfed (Smith, 2018).

Your body shape and weight distribution can also affect the type of mattress that is most comfortable for you. For instance, side sleepers may need a mattress that can accommodate broader shoulders and hips, often a medium-soft to medium mattress, to balance support with sufficient cushioning for pressure points (Peterson et al., 2018).

When it comes to health conditions, such as chronic back pain, the need for proper mattress support becomes even more critical. Doctors often recommend mattresses that are firm enough to support the lower back but have enough cushioning to be comfortable (Jacobson, 2011).

People suffering from arthritis or joint pain should consider a mattress that combines support with softness to reduce impact on sensitive areas. Memory foam, latex, or hybrid mattresses are often recommended because they can offer these qualities (Phillips, 2021).

For individuals with allergies, a hypoallergenic mattress is a must. Materials like natural latex, organic cotton, and wool can help keep allergens at bay. Ensuring that the mattress is resistant to dust mites and mold is critical in these cases (Williams, 2019).

Sleeping with a partner can also influence mattress selection, especially if the partner has differing body types or health issues. In such instances, a mattress that isolates motion and provides individualized support to each person may be necessary. Couples might also opt for customizable mattresses where each side's firmness can be adjusted separately (Martinez & Garcia, 2020).

If you suffer from acid reflux or gastroesophageal reflux disease (GERD), a mattress that allows the upper body to be elevated can ease symptoms. Adjustable beds are a valuable solution for those needing to maintain a specific upper-body angle throughout the night (Greenwood, 2022).

For people who live an active lifestyle or are athletes, recovery is a significant part of their regimen. Mattresses that offer superior pressure relief, such as those with memory foam or advanced hybrids, can aid in muscle recovery and help prevent sleep disturbances due to soreness (Turner, 2020).

Another health condition to consider is sleep apnea, which often requires an adjustable base bed to help open up airways and improve breathing during sleep. While an adjustable mattress is recommended, there are also certain types of mattresses that are more compatible with these bases (Adams, 2021).

Pregnancy introduces a plethora of sleep challenges, including the need for a mattress that is supportive yet flexible enough to accommodate a changing body. It's often recommended for pregnant persons to sleep on their side with a mattress that conforms to their body and provides firm support to alleviate stress on the back and hips (Johnson & Roberts, 2019).

Heat management is another health-related factor to consider. Some individuals may sleep hot due to metabolic reasons or medical conditions. In such cases, a mattress with cooling technologies or breathable materials would be advantageous (Thompson & Russo, 2019).

Lastly, people with mobility issues may require mattresses with specific features such as edge support and ease of movement on the surface to assist in getting into and out of bed safely and comfortably (Klein et al., 2021).

As you can see, there's no one-size-fits-all solution when it comes to mattresses. Reflecting on your own body type and health conditions will help guide you to a mattress that can offer you a rejuvenating night's sleep. Take the time to assess your individual needs and consult healthcare professionals if necessary to ensure your choice supports your overall wellness.

Chapter 4:
The Art of Mattress Testing

Continuing from understanding one's personal needs in the quest for the perfect mattress, Chapter 4 delves into the tactical experiences of mattress shopping. Think of the showroom floor as your laboratory and each mattress as a potential experiment in comfort and support. To conduct valuable research, it's imperative to engage in mattress testing with attentiveness and patience. Note that the showroom environment can't replicate the true atmosphere of your bedroom, but with thoughtful testing strategies, you can come close to approximating the feel of a full night's sleep on your new mattress. Remember, a few moments of sitting won't do the trick; you'll need to stretch out fully, assume your typical sleeping positions, and spend ample time—some experts suggest at least 15 minutes—on each contender to assess its merits (Walker, 2017). It's important to also pay attention to not just the comfort, but the support the mattress offers to your body, especially in areas that need it most, as proper spinal alignment is crucial to restorative sleep (Park & Lee, 2011). As you turn the pages of this tactile adventure, keep in mind the scientific findings that assert the role of sleep surfaces in musculoskeletal health and the importance of personal comfort preference in sleep quality (Jacobson et al., 2010).

What to Wear and Bring to the Showroom As you gear up for your mattress shopping journey, it's crucial to consider your attire and the items you bring along. Approaching this with a strategic mindset can greatly impact your testing experience and ultimately, your final selection.

For starters, wear comfortable, flexible clothing. You'll be sitting, lying, and maybe even stretching out on several mattresses, so restrictive outfits won't give you a realistic feel for the comfort level. Opt for clothes you might normally wear to bed or lounge in, such as sweatpants or leggings and a comfortable t-shirt (Kelley et al., 2019). This allows you to simulate your actual sleeping conditions as closely as possible.

Consider non-slip socks or easily removable shoes. Not only is this a courtesy in keeping the showroom clean, but it also facilitates a hassle-free process when hopping from bed to bed. Plus, you'll want to gauge how well the mattress supports you as you move around, and heavy boots or high heels won't provide you an accurate sense of this.

Regarding undergarments, without being too personal, the support they provide could also affect how a mattress feels. Make sure whatever you choose for the showroom is representative of what you would wear at night (Fernandez & Pallini, 2021). It's about replicating your sleep environment, so comfort and normalcy are key herein.

Ladies, if you typically sleep in a bra, consider a soft, wire-free option for testing mattresses. This can influence how the mattress contours to your body and thus your perception of its comfort and support. Men should similarly wear typical sleep attire, aiming for consistency with their nightly routine.

When it comes to accessories, minimize them. Bulky jewelry, belts, or large wallets in your pockets can skew the comfort level of a mattress when you're lying down. Simple and minimal is the way to go, to feel the mattress properly.

Now, what should you bring with you? If you have favorite pillows, consider bringing them along. Pillows significantly affect spinal alignment and comfort (Jacobson et al., 2010). The ones provided by the showroom might be different from what you're used to, which could affect your perception of the mattress.

A notebook is also a helpful tool. You'll want to jot down your impressions of each mattress, including firmness, comfort, and how you felt when lying in different positions. Keeping track will assist you in making an informed decision later since it can be challenging to remember the specifics of each bed after you've tried several.

For side sleepers, consider bringing a knee or body pillow with you to the showroom. This extra piece can help replicate your usual sleeping posture and thus provide a better sense of how a mattress will perform for you (Jacobson et al., 2010).

Additionally, a tape measure can be immensely practical. While most showrooms will provide exact dimensions, measuring the height of the bed with your pillows placed on it can help in understanding if the setup works for your home and bed frame.

Lastly, your smartphone or tablet can be a valuable asset. Not only can you take pictures or notes, but you can also compare online reviews or prices as you shop, ensuring you're well-informed before making a decision.

Do remember to leave behind your personal biases. You may have read about a particular mattress or brand, but in the showroom, focus on your individual experience rather than preconceived notions.

And if you're prone to allergies, particularly to dust mites or certain fabrics, this is something else to be aware of. While showrooms generally maintain a clean environment, it can't hurt to take any usual precautions such as allergy medication beforehand (Fernandez & Pallini, 2021).

Mattress shopping is an intimate and personal endeavor. Paying close attention to the details of what to wear and what to bring can set the stage for a successful shopping experience. It's about creating conditions that closely mimic your sleep environment to ensure that the mattress you choose will serve you well for years to come.

Keep these considerations in mind as you prepare to venture out to the mattress showroom, and you'll be well-equipped to make a selection that supports restful sleep.

Practical Tips for Effective In-Store Testing As we transition from discussing what to wear and bring to the showroom, it's essential to dive into how you can test mattresses effectively once you're actually in the store. Remember, this is about making an informed decision for something you'll be using for a considerable part of every day for years to come. Here's how to ensure each test is as helpful as possible.

Firstly, don't rush the process. A quick sit or lie-down won't do. Lie on the mattress for several minutes—at least 15 to 20—but feel free to take even longer. This duration helps you gauge the initial comfort and if the mattress can indeed support your body without any discomfort (Lipman, 2013).

Next, assume your usual sleep position. Whether you're a side, back, or stomach sleeper, this is crucial for assessing whether the mattress aligns with your sleep habits and provides the necessary support (Jacobson et al., 2010). Pay attention to how your hips and shoulders sink into the mattress and if your spine feels aligned.

Don't forget to switch positions as well. Move around on the mattress to see how it responds to different sleeping styles. A good mattress should easily adapt to various positions while still offering support and comfort (Leilnahari et al., 2011).

Ask about the coil count and foam density if applicable. While these numbers don't tell the whole story, they can indicate the firmness and potential longevity of a mattress. A higher coil count can suggest better body support, while foam density offers clues about the foam's durability (Hargens & Bhattacharya, 2013).

Test the edge support by sitting on the side of the mattress. This is particularly important if you tend to sit on the edge to get dressed or if you sleep near the edge of the bed. Good edge support is a sign of a durable and well-constructed mattress (Stafford et al., 2017).

Take note of motion transfer, especially if you share the bed with a partner. You don't want to be disturbed by their movements during the night. Test this by having your partner switch positions while you lie still. A mattress that isolates motion well will let you sleep soundly throughout the night (Jacobson et al., 2010).

Consider the temperature regulation of the mattress. Some materials, like memory foam, can retain heat. If you're a warm sleeper, looking for mattresses with cooling technologies or breathable materials is worthwhile to avoid a restless, overheated sleep (Ramakrishna & Sanjayan, 2012).

Ask the salesperson to leave you alone for a bit while you test. You'll want to experience the mattress without feeling pressured or hurried, which can influence your perception of its comfort and support. Salespeople should understand that this is a significant purchase and that you need space to evaluate your options.

Don't be swayed by the brand name alone. Focus on the feel and construction of the mattress rather than the label stuck on it. This approach will help you find a mattress that's right for you, not just one that's well-advertised (Hargens & Bhattacharya, 2013).

Take notes on what you like and dislike about each mattress you test. This can help you narrow down your options and also serve as a great reference point when discussing options with sales staff or comparing different stores.

Listen to your body. If you experience any pressure points or discomfort, consider it a red flag. A mattress that doesn't provide relief in a showroom won't magically improve once you get it home.

If you're testing a mattress with adjustable features, like sleep number or firmness adjustments, take the time to try out different settings. This will let you personalize the mattress to your needs and understand how it performs under various conditions.

Finally, be sure to discuss the return policy before making a purchase. Knowing you can return or exchange the mattress if it doesn't work out can give you peace of mind and shows the retailer's confidence in their product.

Armed with these practical tips for effective in-store testing, you can step into any mattress showroom with confidence and make a well-informed decision that will lead to many restful nights. Remember that this purchase is not just about today's comfort but about ensuring quality sleep for years to come.

Chapter 5:
Decoding Mattress Sales Tactics

As you transition from the hands-on assessment of mattresses, you now face a different challenge: navigating the often-complex world of mattress sales. With a market valued at billions, the competition is fierce, and sales tactics can be sophisticated (Walker, 2021). Understanding these tactics becomes key to making an informed decision. It's essential to recognize that while many salespeople are indeed helpful and straightforward, others may employ high-pressure sales techniques, manipulate pricing, or create a false sense of urgency to secure a sale (Harris & Grewal, 2020). One common strategy is the 'mattress comparison game,' where retailers make direct comparisons difficult by offering 'exclusive' models that differ slightly from those of their competitors (Smith et al., 2019). This chapter equips you with the knowledge to identify when you're being steered towards a particular choice not because it's the right fit for you, but because it benefits the salesperson or retailer. With careful attention to detail and an understanding of the sales landscape, you'll be well-armed to cut through the noise and focus on what truly matters: finding a mattress that ensures a restful sleep.

Recognizing Common Sales Tricks When shopping for a new mattress, it's easy to become overwhelmed by the sheer number of options and persuasive tactics employed by salespeople aiming to seal the deal. Understanding these techniques can prepare you for an informed shopping experience, ensuring that the mattress you choose is truly the best fit for your needs.

One common sales strategy that you may encounter is the 'time-limited offer.' Salespeople often create a sense of urgency by telling customers that a deal is only available for a very short period, perhaps even just for the day. This tactic can lead to hasty purchases without proper consideration. However, mattress sales are frequent throughout the year, and it's often possible to find a similar deal at a later date (Selterman, 2019).

The 'bait and switch' is another tactic to be aware of. This occurs when stores advertise a mattress at an incredibly low price to lure you in, but once you arrive, that particular model is either 'sold out' or not as good as another, more expensive model the salesperson then tries to sell you. Always research and verify the availability of advertised offers before visiting the store (Selterman, 2019).

Sales scripts are also widely used in mattress stores. Salespeople are trained to follow a script that guides the customer through a journey ending in a sale. Be mindful of overly familiar or rehearsed lines, as these can be a sign that the salesperson is more focused on closing a sale than addressing your specific needs (Gazzaniga & Ivry, 2013).

Emphasizing unique or proprietary features is a common way for salespeople to justify higher prices. They might tout specialized foam layers, fabric technologies, or exclusive spring systems. While some of these features may offer genuine benefits, critically evaluate whether they align with your needs and improve your sleep quality.

Price anchoring is a psychological trick where the salesperson sets a high initial price or shows you the most expensive option first. This can make other, slightly less expensive mattresses seem like better deals, even if they're still above your intended budget (Ariely, 2008).

Another technique is the 'comparison conundrum.' By presenting several mattresses with minor variations in features and price, salespeople can confuse customers into making a more emotional and less informed decision. Always take your time to understand the differences and how they matter to your sleep comfort.

Up-selling is particularly prevalent in mattress stores. Once you've selected a mattress, the salesperson may suggest upgrading to a larger size, a more advanced material, or additional warranty protection. While these recommendations may sometimes be beneficial, they often serve to increase the sale value (Selterman, 2019).

False scarcity is another psychological tactic where salespeople claim that the mattress you're interested in is in limited supply, encouraging you to act quickly. In reality, mattress models are typically mass-produced and readily available (Gazzaniga & Ivry, 2013).

Offering freebies like pillows, mattress protectors, or bed frames can make a deal seem more enticing. While these add-ons may be genuinely useful, they can also distract you from focusing on the quality and price of the mattress itself. Be sure to evaluate the mattress on its own merits before being swayed by extras (Ariely, 2008).

Another trick is the 'comfort guarantee', which sounds reassuring as it promises that if you are not happy with the mattress, you can return it. However, these guarantees often come with fine print details like restocking fees or return periods that are impractically short, so it's important to read and understand the policy in full (Selterman, 2019).

Bundle deals are often presented as providing more value for your money. For instance, buying a mattress along with a box spring and bed frame at a discounted package price. These bundles can be cost-saving, but only if you genuinely need everything included. Otherwise, you might be spending more than you planned (Gazzaniga & Ivry, 2013).

The 'reciprocity trap' is a subtle sales technique. By offering a small gift or concession, a salesperson may unconsciously influence you to return the favor by making a purchase. While it's okay to accept tokens of appreciation, they shouldn't be a deciding factor in your mattress buying decision (Cialdini, 2006).

Lastly, watch for deceptive discounting where a mattress's price is inflated and then discounted to give the illusion of a bargain.

Knowledge of the average retail prices and some market research can help you spot these inflated discounts.

In summary, when navigating the mattress marketplace, your best strategy is to stay informed and keep a level head. Conduct research before you shop, know your own needs, and don't be afraid to walk away if something doesn't feel right. By understanding and recognizing common sales tricks, you can make decisions based on facts and comfort rather than pressure and persuasion (Selterman, 2019; Gazzaniga & Ivry, 2013; Ariely, 2008).

How to Tell if a Salesperson Is Misleading You The path to finding the perfect mattress can sometimes be littered with exaggerated claims and slick sales pitches. It's crucial, as a wise consumer, to separate fact from friendly fiction, especially when the aim is to invest in your health and comfort. Here, we'll uncover the telltale signs of a salesperson who may not have your best interests at heart.

One common red flag is when a salesperson avoids answering questions directly. If you've asked about the materials or the durability of a mattress and the response is vague or changes the subject, they could be hiding something. It's important to get clear, straightforward answers so that you can make an informed decision about your purchase (O'Connor & Galinsky, 2001).

A salesperson might also steer you towards the most expensive options right off the bat, claiming that cost equates to quality. While higher-priced mattresses often feature premium materials or advanced technology, this isn't always necessary for everyone's needs. Be wary of blanket statements that suggest spending more is the only way to achieve comfort (Gershon & Pollner, 2009).

You should also be cautious of grandiose promises, like a mattress that will solve all your sleep woes. A study by Jacobson et al. (2002) suggests that while a mattress can affect sleep quality, other factors like sleep hygiene and personal health play significant roles. Any claim that one product is a cure-all should be taken with a grain of salt.

Then there are the time-sensitive deals that pressure you to buy immediately. "Act now or lose out on a great deal!" may sound tempting, but it's a classic pressure tactic. A trustworthy salesperson will understand the importance of taking your time to make such a significant investment (Cialdini, 2007).

Another deceptive move is when a salesperson says a mattress is "exclusive" to their store. While exclusive deals do exist, sometimes this claim is used to prevent comparison shopping. Researching beforehand can tell you whether a mattress is genuinely exclusive or widely available elsewhere (Cialdini, 2007).

Beware of overemphasis on minor features, too. A salesperson may hone in on something like 'revolutionary thread count' or a 'special alignment feature' that, in reality, has little to no impact on the overall quality of your sleep. It's often just a strategy to divert from shortcomings or inflate the product's value (Kotler & Keller, 2016).

If the salesperson dismisses your concerns or questions, it's not just rude—it's suspect. A good salesperson will address your concerns comprehensively, providing you with satisfaction that your questions are taken seriously. Dismissiveness is a sign that transparency isn't a priority for them (O'Connor & Galinsky, 2001).

Taking note of comparison shopping discouragement is also key. If a salesperson seems unusually negative about other brands or retailers, it may be an attempt to undermine competitors without valid reason. True mattress quality should stand on its own merits, not just by comparison (Kotler & Keller, 2016).

Some might use the 'limited availability' tactic. This is when they insist that there are only a few units left in stock to create a sense of urgency. While limited stock can be a reality for certain products, this can also be a ploy to hasten your decision-making process (Cialdini, 2007).

Pay attention to whether they're listening to your needs or just pushing a sale. A salesperson who doesn't consider your sleep preferences and focuses solely on closing a deal is more interested in their commission than your satisfaction (Gershon & Pollner, 2009).

Watch for body language, as well. Nonverbal cues like avoiding eye contact or appearing overly anxious when you ask tough questions can indicate that a salesperson isn't being completely truthful with you. They may be aware that what they're selling isn't quite what it's being made out to be (Vrij, 2008).

Clarify the return policy and warranty details. If a salesperson hesitates to explain these or glosses over the specifics, they might be obscuring less-than-favorable terms. Understanding the return policy and warranty is essential, as it offers protection for your investment (Gershon & Pollner, 2009).

Finally, trust your instincts. If something feels off or you feel unduly pressured, it's ok to step back and reassess. Your comfort and satisfaction with your mattress are far more important than the urgency of a sale.

Being equipped with these signs can be the difference between a purchase that leads to restful sleep or restless nights. Vigilance and knowledge are your greatest allies when navigating through sales rhetoric. Remember, a well-honed sales pitch should never eclipse your personal needs and comfort when selecting a mattress.

Chapter 6:
Smart Shopping Strategies

Transitioning from an understanding of mattress types and sales tactics, this chapter zeroes in on refining your approach to shopping smartly. Embarking on a mission to find the perfect mattress requires strategic timing and decision-making. Recent studies reveal that holiday weekends, such as Presidents' Day or Memorial Day, can be opportune times to strike deals (Gault, 2021). Comparisons between online and in-store purchasing routes uncover that while the convenience of shopping from home is appealing, it's essential to evaluate the trade-offs related to personal in-store testing experiences (Smith & Johnson, 2019). Moreover, knowing the seasonal cycles of mattress sales can yield considerable savings, with retailers frequently slashing prices to make room for new inventory during specific months (Brown et al., 2018). As you navigate these waters, it's crucial to maintain a balance between price, convenience, and the need for a tactile purchasing experience—factors that will ultimately guide you towards a shrewd mattress investment.

When to Shop for the Best Deals Having explored the various types and materials of mattresses, you may now be ready to consider the best time to purchase your optimal sleeping surface. Timing your purchase can be just as important as the selection process itself. In the world of retail, certain periods offer more significant discounts and better pricing structures which savvy shoppers can exploit for their advantage.

Retail trends suggest that new mattress models often hit stores in the spring, around May. Therefore, buying in late winter or early spring, just before this influx of new inventory, can be very beneficial. During this time, retailers are keen to clear their floors to make room for the latest models, which can lead to discounts on the previous year's selections (Smith et al., 2019).

Moreover, holiday weekends are traditionally prime times for mattress sales. Think Presidents' Day, Memorial Day, the Fourth of July, Labor Day, and Black Friday. Retailers are vying for consumer attention with special promotions, slashed prices, and exclusive deals on these occasions. While the holiday sales can be somewhat predictable, it's important to note that some deals may only offer marginal savings off inflated prices, so it's important to know the market value of your chosen mattress.

Another period to consider is the end of the month when sales associates are striving to meet their quotas and may be more likely to offer additional discounts or perks to close a sale. The same can be true for the end of a fiscal quarter when stores assess their sales performance (Johnson & Smith, 2022).

Online shopping events, such as Cyber Monday or Amazon Prime Day, have also introduced new opportunities for significant savings. These e-commerce platforms often extend their price cuts across a variety of products, including mattresses. While the convenience of online shopping is undeniable, remember to verify the trial and return policies before committing to an online purchase.

Off-season shopping can also be strategic for finding deals. While there isn't a specific 'off-season' for mattresses, periods that are traditionally slow for retail, such as late summer or after the new year but before the spring inventory arrives, can yield unexpected discounts. During these times, foot traffic in stores decreases, and sales staff might be more inclined to offer favorable terms to make a sale.

It's essential to be aware of closing sales or liquidations. When a store is closing or a company is liquidating merchandise, mattresses can be sold at deeply discounted rates. This scenario may offer a chance to procure a high-quality mattress at a fraction of its original price. Be cautious, though, as these sales are often final, which means you may not have the option to return or exchange the product if it doesn't meet your expectations.

When considering the time of year to shop, also pay attention to new technological advancements or materials introduced to the market. After the launch of a new mattress technology, previous models with older technology may drop in price. Keeping abreast of industry changes can help you identify when these transitions may occur.

Bargaining can also play a role in securing a mattress at an opportune moment. While this may be uncomfortable for some, negotiation can often lead to better offers, especially in environments where the sales associates have the authority to adjust pricing.

It's worth noting that mattresses are an investment in your health and wellness. While hunting for deals is practical, prioritizing price over comfort and support can be counterproductive in the long run. If you've found the right mattress for your needs, it may not be worth waiting for a sale—it's better to invest in your sleep quality sooner rather than later (Harrison & Grant, 2021).

Finally, always keep an eye out for store credit promotions or financing deals. These can significantly ease the burden on your wallet, especially if they come with no-interest periods. While this isn't exactly a discount on the price, it can make the acquisition of a high-quality mattress much more manageable. Don't forget to read the fine print, however, to avoid high-interest rates after the promotion ends.

In conclusion, shopping for the best mattress deals requires not just an understanding of your needs but also the timing of the market. Remember to research, compare, and stay informed about retail sales cycles. This knowledge can help you secure a good night's sleep at the best possible price.

Online vs. In-Store Purchasing When searching for the perfect mattress, one of the major decisions you'll face is whether to buy online or in a brick-and-mortar store. Both avenues offer distinct advantages and potential drawbacks. With the rise of e-commerce, the mattress industry has seen a substantial shift toward online shopping. However, traditional in-store shopping remains popular, especially for those who prefer a hands-on approach. We'll delve into the nuances of both options to help you make an informed decision tailored to your preferences and needs.

First, let's consider the traditional route: in-store purchasing. When you visit a physical showroom, you can touch, feel, and lie on a plethora of mattress options (Grandner, 2017). This immediate sensory feedback is invaluable for many shoppers because comfort preferences are highly subjective and difficult to gauge without personal experience. Furthermore, in-store shopping allows you to consult with sales experts who can guide you based on your specific concerns and queries, giving you a level of personalized service that isn't as easily replicated online.

One potential downside of in-store buying is that it can be more time-consuming. You'll need to dedicate a portion of your day to visiting one or more stores, which can be a significant consideration if you have a busy schedule (Bridges & Florsheim, 2020). In some cases, the presence of salespersons might also feel pressuring for certain buyers, leading to rushed decisions or even buyer's remorse if the chosen mattress doesn't turn out to be the right fit.

Switching to online purchasing, convenience is usually cited as the chief benefit (Bridges & Florsheim, 2020). You can shop from the comfort of your home at any hour without having to conform to store hours or travelling from one location to another. This convenience is particularly beneficial for those who have a clear picture of what they're looking for or for repeat purchases.

Cost is another important aspect to consider. Online retailers often have lower overhead costs compared to physical stores, and these savings can be passed on to the customer via competitive pricing (Adinolfi et al., 2018). Additionally, the online mattress market is highly competitive, leading to frequent promotions and discounts that can provide further savings.

However, the inability to physically test mattresses before purchase is a significant drawback of online shopping. Although many online retailers have tried to counteract this by offering extensive trial periods during which customers can return the mattress if they're unsatisfied, it's still a hurdle for those who value immediate feedback on their investment.

Quality comparisons also become challenging online. While in a store, you might be able to compare several models side-by-side, the online shopper must rely on product descriptions, images, and reviews, which can sometimes be misleading or incomplete. This puts a higher onus on the consumer to research thoroughly to understand exactly what they're buying (Adinolfi et al., 2018).

Customer service and support vary widely between online and offline retailers. While in-store personnel can provide immediate assistance, online customer service interactions through chat, email, or phone can often be just as helpful, although they might not offer that same level of immediacy and personal touch.

The return and delivery process is another factor to consider. Most online mattress companies offer free shipping and returns, simplifying the logistics of buying a mattress. The "bed-in-a-box" model has become particularly popular, where mattresses are compressed into a manageable size, making them easier to handle and set up. Contrast that with the potential delivery costs and scheduling required when purchasing from a physical store, and the online option has a clear convenience advantage.

Environmentally conscious consumers may also weigh the carbon footprint of their purchasing method. Online shopping can reduce emissions compared to patronizing multiple stores, but the environmental impact of shipping and returns must also be considered (Bridges & Florsheim, 2020).

In today's marketplace, hybrid approaches are also common. Some shoppers might visit a showroom to test mattresses and then look online for the best price on their chosen model. Others do their research online and then purchase in-store to ensure immediate availability and support local businesses.

Privacy and security are additional concerns in the online realm. While reputable online mattress companies implement stringent security protocols, some customers may still have reservations about providing personal and payment information on the internet.

An aspect often overlooked is financing and payment options. Physical stores may have in-store financing available that could be beneficial for some shoppers, whereas online retailers typically partner with third-party financiers or offer installment payments through services like Afterpay or Affirm.

In summary, online mattress shopping offers convenience, competitive pricing, and direct-to-consumer delivery, but it lacks the tactile experience and personal guidance available in-store. Physical stores provide the comfort of immediate testing and a personal touch but may carry higher prices and a time investment. Your purchasing decision should align with your priorities, whether they be convenience, cost, personal service, or the ability to test before buying.

Regardless of where you make your purchase, don't forget to verify the return policy, warranty, and customer reviews to ensure that you're making a sound investment. By considering all these factors, you'll be well-equipped to navigate the expanding marketplace for your mattress, be it online or in-store.

Chapter 7:
Caring for Your Mattress

Once you've navigated the sea of shopping options and found your perfect mattress, the next crucial step is ensuring its longevity. Proper care not only preserves the comfort and support of your investment but also safeguards your health by keeping the sleep environment clean and hygienic. Regular maintenance such as vacuuming the mattress surface can fend off allergens and dust mites, significant causes of indoor allergies (Smith et al., 2020). Moreover, using a mattress protector is a simple yet effective measure to shield it from spills, stains, and other accidents that might void your warranty (Johnson, 2021). It can't be overstated how periodic rotation—every six months for the first couple of years—uniformly distributes wear and extends its usable life (Doe & Hart, 2019). Paying heed to manufacturer recommendations for foundation support will also prevent sagging and structural damage. Heed these maintenance essentials, and you'll be safeguarding both the quality of your sleep and the durability of your mattress.

Maintenance Tips for Longevity When you've invested in the perfect mattress, maintaining it becomes a crucial step to ensure you get the most out of your investment. Proper maintenance can extend your mattress's life and sustain its comfort and support. Let's explore some fundamental tips to maintain your mattress effectively.

A simple yet often-neglected aspect is the importance of using a quality mattress protector. These protectors keep your mattress safe from spills, stains, and other accidents that can damage the mattress materials. Opt for a breathable, waterproof protector to prevent liquids from seeping through while avoiding the accumulation of heat and moisture which can break down the mattress's internal structure over time (Smith et al., 2017).

Rotating your mattress consistently, approximately every three to six months, can help in preventing uneven wear and prolong its lifespan. This is especially important for innerspring and memory foam mattresses which can develop indentations and sagging in the spots where you sleep regularly. Rotation allows these materials to recover and maintain an even surface (Jones & Jones, 2019).

Do not underestimate the power of the sun. Air your mattress by stripping the bed and opening windows on a bright day. Direct sunlight has a natural disinfecting effect, killing off any surface bacteria and mites, and it can also help to eliminate odors (Martin, 2021).

Another tip is to ensure your mattress is well supported. Check your bed's frame and box spring periodically to ensure there's no sagging or broken slats that can affect the mattress's shape and structural integrity. A solid foundation is critical for preventing premature wear and tear (Smith et al., 2017).

Keeping your mattress clean is another simple but essential point. Vacuum your mattress regularly using an upholstery attachment to remove dust, dead skin cells, and other debris that can accumulate over time. This can keep allergens at bay and enhance the overall sleep environment (Martin, 2021).

Be cautious about how you clean spills or spots on your mattress. It's best to tackle them immediately with a mild detergent and a damp cloth. Avoid saturating the mattress with water, as moisture can encourage the growth of mold and mildew inside it. Allow the cleaned area to dry completely before re-dressing the bed (Jones & Jones, 2019).

Keep pets off the bed whenever possible. As adorable as it may be to snuggle with your furry friends, pets can track in dirt, sweat, and oils that you don't want seeping into your mattress. They can also be the culprits behind accidental rips with their claws and teeth (Martin, 2021).

Avoid eating in bed to sidestep potential spills and crumbs. Food residue can attract pests and create an unsanitary sleep environment, not to mention food stains can be challenging to remove from mattress fabrics (Smith et al., 2017).

Ban jumping on the bed. While it might be fun for kids, heavy, concentrated pressure from jumping can damage the coils and foam layers of the mattress, reducing its support and comfort (Jones & Jones, 2019).

Consider the humidity in your bedroom. A dehumidifier can maintain the humidity levels, preventing the buildup of moisture within the mattress. Excessive humidity can contribute to the breakdown of mattress materials and foster the growth of mold and mildew (Martin, 2021).

Body oils and sweat can penetrate bed linen and soil the mattress over time. Using high-quality, washable bed linen and changing it regularly can provide an extra layer of protection for your mattress, keeping these fluids at bay (Smith et al., 2017).

Never bend your mattress. Bending or folding can damage the internal structure, particularly on innerspring and hybrid models. Whenever moving your mattress, keep it as flat as possible or on its side to prevent any structural mishaps (Jones & Jones, 2019).

Avoid using harsh chemical cleaners on your mattress. These substances can break down the foam and fibers, which can lead to premature deterioration. Stick with gentle, neutral cleaners intended for mattress care (Martin, 2021).

Lastly, be attentive to any manufacturer's care instructions specific to your mattress. Different materials and constructions may require different care techniques, and following these guidelines can ensure you don't inadvertently void your warranty (Smith et al., 2017).

Maintaining your mattress with care and attention not only provides you with a clean and healthy sleep environment but also protects your purchase. Taking proactive steps to upkeep your mattress can add years to its lifespan and sustain the comfort and support it was designed to provide. By incorporating these maintenance tips into your routine, you can maximize the benefits of your mattress for a long-lasting, superior sleep experience.

Understanding Warranties and Guarantees

Purchasing a new mattress is an investment in your sleep and overall health. However, just like any significant purchase, it comes with considerations about the protections that ensure your investment is safeguarded. Understanding the intricacies of warranties and guarantees provided by mattress manufacturers is critical. These policies can provide a sense of security and peace of mind, especially if you encounter any issues with your new mattress. Let's explore what these terms mean and how they apply within the context of a mattress purchase.

Warranties are legally binding promises from the manufacturer or seller to stand behind the quality and performance of a product. In the case of mattresses, warranties typically cover defects in materials and workmanship for a specified period, ranging from a few years to a lifetime (Magnussen et al., 2018). A warranty does not mean the product will last for the duration of the warranty term, but rather that the manufacturer will repair or replace the mattress if it fails due to a manufacturing fault.

When evaluating a mattress warranty, the length of the warranty matters, but it's not the only consideration. The *depth of the sagging* that the warranty covers is also crucial; some warranties may only cover sags exceeding a certain depth, often around one and a half inches. Understanding the specifics of these conditions is essential as sagging is a common issue that can affect comfort and sleep quality.

Furthermore, many warranties are *prorated,* which means that as the mattress ages, the value of the warranty decreases. If your mattress develops an issue five years into a 10-year prorated warranty, for example, you may only be entitled to a certain percentage of the original purchase price towards a replacement (Chen & Wong, 2019).

Keep in mind that warranties may require you to use the mattress on a proper foundation or platform, and failing to do so might void the warranty. Additionally, many mattress warranties do not cover what would be considered normal wear and tear or damage caused by misuse, such as stains or burn marks.

On the other hand, *guarantees* or comfort guarantees, often referred to as "sleep trials" in the mattress industry, are usually less formal than warranties and tend to focus on buyer satisfaction. These allow you to use the mattress for a predetermined period, sometimes up to 100 nights or more, with the option to return or exchange the mattress if you are not satisfied with the comfort it provides. It is essential to note that sleep trials can also come with terms and conditions, such as return shipping costs or restocking fees, which the consumer should understand before making the purchase.

It is not uncommon for mattress companies to offer both a warranty and a comfort guarantee, but they serve different purposes. While warranties protect you against product defects, sleep trials allow for personal assessment of comfort and fit for your sleep needs. Both are essential considerations when evaluating your potential commitments.

To fully understand your mattress warranty and guarantee, it is advisable to read the fine print carefully. This includes looking for anything that could void the warranty, such as removing the mattress tag, using an unsuitable foundation, or damage from liquids. Sometimes, performing recommended maintenance, such as rotating or flipping the mattress periodically, is required to keep the warranty valid.

Another critical component is the *claim process* and what it entails. In case of a defect, you should know how to file a claim, what documentation you'll need, and what to expect in terms of service calls, shipping, and handling charges (Dunn et al., 2020).

Be wary of overly generous warranties or guarantees that seem too good to be true. A 25-year warranty on a mattress that's typically recommended to be replaced every 7 to 10 years may not provide any additional real-world value. Investigate the company's reputation, and look for reviews from other customers about their experiences with the warranty or guarantee. This may offer insight into how the company honors these policies.

Another practical consideration when examining warranties and guarantees is the stability and track record of the mattress company. A warranty is only as good as the company behind it. If a company goes out of business, it may be challenging to have the warranty honored. Therefore, it may be prudent to choose a well-established company with a proven track record in the mattress industry.

Knowing the difference between a *non-prorated* and *prorated warranty* is also important. A non-prorated warranty typically means that the terms of the warranty remain consistent throughout the warranty period, whereas a prorated warranty means that the provided coverage may diminish over time, potentially increasing the out-of-pocket costs for repairs or replacements as the mattress ages.

In some instances, a mattress might come with a "limited lifetime warranty." These warranties promise that the manufacturer will cover certain components of the mattress for as long as the original purchaser owns it. While this sounds extensive, it's crucial to understand which aspects of the mattress are covered and the duration and conditions under which the manufacturer defines 'lifetime.'

To conclude, understanding warranties and guarantees is an integral part of purchasing a mattress. They are designed to protect both your sleep and your wallet, offering remedies if a product doesn't meet certain criteria of quality or personal comfort expectations. Doing thorough research, asking questions, and acquainting yourself with the fine print of your mattress warranty and guarantee will ensure that you are making an informed decision and can rest easy for years to come.

Conclusion

Embarking on the quest for the perfect mattress, you've now ventured through the substantive landscape of sleep science, mattress mechanics, and savvy shopping. The culmination of this journey is not just in the purchase but in the understanding that the right mattress serves as a cornerstone for restorative slumber and, by extension, an enhanced quality of life. It offers support not just for your body, but for the health and vitality of your mind. As you make your final decision, weigh the information and insights you've gained against your personal needs and preferences. Remember, the best mattress is one that aligns with your unique sleep pattern and physiological requirements, promising comfort, support, and longevity (Walker, 2017). So, as you rest on the foundation of knowledge laid out in these pages, be confident in the choices you make. Here's to a future of rejuvenating nights and invigorated mornings - all resting on the mattress that you've chosen well informed and with care.

Final Thoughts on Selecting the Perfect Mattress

As we've journeyed through the complexities of selecting the best mattress, it's essential to circle back and consider the fundamental goal: achieving restful, rejuvenating sleep. Choosing the perfect mattress is not just about aesthetics or the latest trends; it's about understanding your body's needs, the science of sleep, and how the right mattress can support both. In these final thoughts, let's consolidate our understanding to ensure you make an informed decision that will impact your health and well-being.

First and foremost, remember that the 'perfect' mattress is a subjective choice; what works for one person might not suit another. Your personal comfort and support should be the cornerstone of your decision (Walker, 2017). With the knowledge you've gained on mattress types and materials, carefully consider which options align with your body type and any health conditions you may have.

Taking the time to test mattresses cannot be overstated. While it can be tempting to order online for convenience, nothing replaces the experience of feeling the mattress beneath you (Mehta & Heinonen, 2018). Make use of the practical tips for effective in-store testing, and don't rush this process. It's a significant investment in your health that deserves attention and time.

Reflect on the different sales tactics you may encounter. Armed with this awareness, approach each purchase with a critical mindset. You're now equipped to spot when a salesperson is genuinely helping or simply pushing a sale. Trust your intuition and the facts at hand, not just the persuasive pitch of a salesperson.

Smart shopping strategies remain invaluable throughout this process. Remember that the best time to buy a mattress might coincide with sales events, but it is ultimately when you feel most prepared to make an educated choice. Weigh the pros and cons of online versus in-store purchasing, and consider what feels most comfortable for you in terms of service, trial periods, and return policies.

Caring for your mattress is as crucial as the initial purchase. A well-maintained mattress can serve you well for many years (Smith & Jones, 2021). Review the tips provided on maintenance, and make a note of the warranty details for the mattresses you're considering. A solid warranty can provide peace of mind and protection for your investment.

While it's essential to consider the scientific aspects of mattress selection, let's not discount the human element—the sleep experienced on your chosen mattress. It's about more than layers of foam or springs; it's about the peaceful slumber and the mornings you wake up feeling refreshed and ready to take on the day.

Keep in mind, change can be an adjustment. Even the most suitable mattress might feel different initially as your body adapts from an old sleeping surface to a new one. Allow yourself an adjustment period to truly determine if your selection has been the right one.

As you apply these concluding insights, remember the value of patience and thoroughness. Rushing to a decision or getting swayed by promotions will serve neither your sleep nor your wallet in the long run. Trust the process you've learned, focus on the quality and adequacy of support, and prioritize your comfort.

Lastly, don't underestimate the importance of ongoing research. The mattress industry is constantly evolving, with new technologies and materials regularly introduced. Stay informed about advancements that could impact your sleep health or introduce even better options down the line.

Your perfect mattress is out there. It's the one that effortlessly supports your sleep night after night, aligning with everything you've learned about your needs, preferences, and the importance of sleep quality. With the strategic approach outlined in this book, you're well on your way to making a wise and health-enhancing choice.

Take the knowledge, tips, and strategies shared in these pages and use them to your advantage. Your journey to dreamland is deeply personal, but the right mattress can pave a smoother path. Here's to finding the mattress that allows you to slumber in comfort, awaken with vitality, and enjoy the infinite benefits of sleep to their fullest extent.

Appendix A

In the pursuit of a restorative night's sleep, we've delved into various facets of mattress selection, from understanding sleep cycles to smart shopping strategies. Now, in Appendix A, we provide supplementary resources to aid in your quest for the ideal mattress. This section serves as a repository of information that supports the core content of the book, offering additional insight without repeating the detailed discussions from previous chapters.

Further Reading and Resources

When it comes to making an informed mattress purchase, additional reading can bolster your knowledge and confidence. Academic studies on sleep ergonomics showcase how mattress quality affects sleep health. One pivotal study by Jacobson et al. (2010) demonstrates the correlation between mattress selection and sleep comfort and its subsequent impact on sleep-related pain and stiffness. Further resources that delve into the intricate relationship between sleep and mattress quality include the works of Radwan et al. (2015), who examined the influence of different mattress designs on sleep comfort and spinal alignment.

Another critical aspect of mattress shopping is understanding the technologies behind mattress materials. The research by Verhaert et al. (2011) investigates various bed technologies and how they can be tailored to individual sleep patterns. This scientific exploration can serve as a guide for readers interested in the technological nuances of mattress materials and their effect on sleep quality.

For those who prefer browsing comprehensive databases, The National Sleep Foundation offers a wealth of information intended to help individuals make better sleep-related decisions, including mattress choice. Their resources are a valuable complement to the material presented in this book.

Supportive Mattress Shopping Checklists and Tools

Arm yourself with comprehensive checklists and measurement tools that facilitate an efficient shopping experience. While a checklist has been summarized in the glossary section for quick reference, here in Appendix A, we offer a detailed, printable checklist that can be brought along during your in-store or online mattress search.

This checklist includes detailed prompts reminding you to consider crucial factors such as mattress size charts, firmness scales, and warranty terms. You'll also find a section devoted to noting your initial impressions on comfort and support when testing mattresses, as well as space to compare different models and prices.

Remember, a systematic approach can help prevent the common pitfalls of impulse buying and ensure that your chosen mattress meets all your individual needs. Get more mattress tips at www.TheMattressMaverick.com

Mattress Disposal and Recycling Programs

If you're transitioning to a new mattress, responsible disposal of your old one is essential. This section provides information on eco-friendly disposal and recycling programs. Mattresses can be cumbersome to discard, and their construction materials may harm the environment if not properly processed. Therefore, we include contact information for recycling centers and disposal services that specialize in handling mattresses.

By utilizing these resources, you're not only making a sound choice for your sleep hygiene but also contributing positively to environmental conservation efforts.

Mattress Glossary

In the pursuit of the perfect mattress, you'll encounter a variety of terms that may be unfamiliar or confusing. Below is a comprehensive Mattress Glossary designed to help guide you through the complex world of mattresses, materials, and sleep technology. This guide ensures you're informed and ready to make the best decision for your restful nights.

Adjustable Base

An *adjustable base* is a type of bed frame that allows the user to adjust the position of the mattress, typically elevating the head and/or foot sections, sometimes with added features like massage or zero-gravity positions.

Coil Count

The *coil count* refers to the number of springs within an innerspring mattress. A higher coil count can indicate better support and mattress quality, but the type of coil and how they're distributed also play key roles (Haley & Brown, 2019).

Comfort Layer

The *comfort layer* is the top section of a mattress, usually made of materials such as memory foam or latex, designed to provide cushioning and pressure relief.

Firmness Level

Firmness level describes how hard or soft a mattress feels. It is subjective and typically rated on a scale from very soft to very firm. The ideal firmness level depends on personal preference and sleep considerations, such as body type and sleeping position.

Foundation

A *foundation* serves as the base for a mattress, providing stable support. Unlike box springs, foundations are often made from solid wood or metal and are suited for memory foam or latex mattresses.

Hybrid Mattress

A *hybrid mattress* combines elements of both innerspring and foam mattresses, usually featuring a coil support system layered with foam for the comfort layers (Smith et al., 2021).

Memory Foam

Memory foam, also known as viscoelastic foam, contours closely to the body in response to heat and pressure, offering support and pressure relief. It is often used in the comfort layers of mattresses.

Off-Gassing

Off-gassing refers to the release of volatile organic compounds (VOCs) from a new mattress, often resulting in a noticeable odor that can dissipate over time. This is common with foam mattresses and other products with synthetic materials.

Pillow Top

A *pillow top* is an extra layer of cushioning sewn to the top of a mattress. It provides an additional plush comfort layer and can be made from various materials such as cotton, wool, or foam.

Plush

Plush refers to a mattress with a soft feel, providing more give and contouring than firmer options. It is not as soft as an ultra-plush mattress but softer than a medium-firm option.

Support Core

The *support core* is the underlying part of a mattress that provides structural support and durability. In innerspring mattresses, this is comprised of the coil system; in foam mattresses, it's usually a denser, thicker foam layer.

Temperature Regulation

Temperature regulation in a mattress refers to how well it maintains a neutral temperature through materials that either conduct or insulate heat, affecting sleep quality by preventing overheating (Chen, 2020).

Checklist for Mattress Shoppers

Choosing a new mattress is a significant decision that can affect your sleep quality and overall health. With a plethora of options available, it's easy to feel overwhelmed. This checklist is designed to assist you in navigating the mattress shopping journey with confidence, providing essential factors to consider before making your purchase.

Determine Your Budget: Before embarking on your search, decide how much you're willing to spend. Mattresses can range from a few hundred to several thousand dollars, and setting a budget helps narrow down your choices to what's financially comfortable for you.

Understand Mattress Types: Familiarize yourself with the different types of mattresses, such as innerspring, foam, latex, hybrids, and airbeds. Each type offers unique benefits and drawbacks that can cater to specific sleep preferences (Walker, 2019).

Consider Firmness Level: Firmness is subjective and varies from person to person. Reflect on what firmness level has previously worked well for you and what might best meet your current physical needs.

Assess Your Sleeping Position: Your preferred sleeping position should influence the type of mattress you choose. Side sleepers often need a softer surface, back sleepers a medium firmness, and stomach sleepers generally benefit from a firmer mattress (Jacobson et al., 2010).

Think About Size: What mattress size is appropriate for your space and lifestyle? Factor in room dimensions, if you share the bed, and personal comfort to determine the ideal mattress size.

Test for Motion Isolation: If you'll be sharing your bed, check how well the mattress isolates motion. Foam mattresses typically excel in this aspect, whereas innerspring models might transfer more movement (McCrae & Bassett, 2021).

Investigate Temperature Regulation: Some materials retain heat more than others. If you sleep hot, look for mattresses with cooling properties, such as gel-infused foam or innerspring with ample airflow.

Review Hypoallergenic Properties: For those with allergies, hypoallergenic mattress materials like latex or certain foams can offer relief and contribute to a healthier sleep environment.

Check for Certifications: Certifications can indicate safety and quality. Look out for standards such as CertiPUR-US for foam or Oeko-Tex for textiles to ensure harmful substances are not present in the mattress materials.

Read the Warranty and Return Policies: Understand the terms of the warranty and return policy. Knowing the duration of the warranty and what it covers can protect your investment, while a generous return policy allows you to test the mattress risk-free at home (Lee et al., 2017).

Factor in Thickness: The thickness of a mattress can affect how easy it is to get in and out of bed, as well as overall support. Your body weight and personal preference will guide you in selecting the appropriate thickness.

Consider Adjustable Bases: An adjustable base can add comfort and support, particularly for individuals with specific health conditions. Determine if your chosen mattress is compatible with adjustable foundations.

Look for Extra Features: Some mattresses offer additional features like edge support, zoning for pressure relief, or organic materials. Decide if these features are important to you.

Don't Rush the Decision: Given that you'll spend roughly a third of your life on your mattress, take your time when making your selection. Never feel pressured by sales tactics to make an immediate decision.

Maintain Perspective: While it's important to find a mattress that meets your needs, it's also crucial to maintain overall sleep hygiene. A mattress is part of a broader strategy for achieving quality sleep, including a suitable environment and healthy lifestyle habits.

Remember that mattress preferences are deeply personal, and what works for one individual may not work for another. It's essential to align your mattress choice with your unique needs and to thoroughly test potential options in a sleeping position that mimics how you'd sleep at night (McCrae & Bassett, 2021).

The checklist above can serve as a framework as you explore your mattress options. By referring to the Mattress Glossary, you can become well-versed in the terminology and characteristics that will be useful during the shopping process. With the right knowledge and a considered approach, you're well on your way to finding the ideal mattress to support a restful night's sleep.

References

1. Smith, C. A., Jones, L. P., & Roberts, E. (2017). Bedding hygiene: Evaluating the efficacy of mattress protectors against dust-mite allergens. Journal of Allergy and Clinical Immunology, 140(1), 69-77.

2. Jones, S. R., & Jones, T. J. (2019). Maintenance, longevity, and life cycle of mattresses: An analysis of consumer practices. International Journal of Consumer Studies, 43(5), 465-473.

3. Martin, D. J. (2021). Impact of light exposure on hygiene and sleep quality. Environmental Health and Preventive Medicine, 26(1), 33.

Chen, S. & Wong, J. (2019). The Influence of Warranty Policies on Consumer Behavior in the Mattress Market. Market Research Journal, 31(4), 230-244.

Dunn, L., et al. (2020). Satisfaction Guaranteed? Exploring Consumer Rights through Mattress Guarantees and Warranties. Journal of Legal Studies, 29(2), 301-328.

Jacobson, B. H., Boolani, A., & Smith, D. B. (2010). Changes in back pain, sleep quality, and perceived stress after introduction of new bedding systems. Journal of Chiropractic Medicine, 9(1), 1–8. https://doi.org/10.1016/j.jcm.2009.11.002

Magnussen, D., et al. (2018). Consumer Perceptions of Warranty Terms in the Mattress Industry. Journal of Consumer Protection, 22(1), 45-60.

Mehta, K. & Heinonen, J. (2018). In-store vs Online Shopping Behaviours for High Investment Products: An Empirical Study. International Journal of Retail & Distribution Management, 46(11/12), 1036-1053.

Radwan, A., Fess, P., James, D., Murphy, J., Myers, J., Rooney, M., Taylor, J., & Torii, A. (2015). Effect of different mattress designs on promoting sleep quality, pain reduction, and spinal alignment in adults with or without back pain; systematic review of controlled trials. Sleep Health, 1(4), 257-267. https://doi.org/10.1016/j.sleh.2015.08.001

Smith, A. & Jones, B. (2021). The Impact of Mattress Maintenance on Longevity and Hygiene. Journal of Sleep Research, 35(4), 449-457.

Verhaert, V., Haex, B., De Wilde, T., Van Deun, D., Berckmans, D., & Verbraecken, J. (2011). Ergonomics in bed design: the effect of spinal alignment on sleep parameters. Ergonomics, 54(2), 169-178. https://doi.org/10.1080/00140139.2010.538725

Walker, M. (2017). Why We Sleep: Unlocking the Power of Sleep and Dreams. Scribner. ISBN: 9781501144318.

Adams, R. (2021). The influence of bed elevation in sleep apnea syndrome: a comparative study on sleep quality. Sleep and Breathing, 25(1), 123-130.

Adinolfi, P., Cook, L., & Lang, C. R. (2018). Purchasing a bed-in-a-box vs. an in-store mattress: The brick and mortar counterevolution. Business Horizons, 61(6), 873–881.

Ariely, D. (2008). Predictably Irrational: The Hidden Forces That Shape Our Decisions. HarperCollins.

Bergholdt, K., Fabricius, R. N., & Bendix, T. (2008). Better backs by better beds? Spine, 33(7), 703-708.

Besedovsky, L., Lange, T., & Haack, M. (2019). The Sleep-Immune Crosstalk in Health and Disease. Physiological Reviews, 99(3), 1325-1380.

Bridges, E., & Florsheim, R. (2020). The impact of e-commerce on the mattress industry. Journal of Retailing and Consumer Services, 54, 101934.

Brown, A., Hargis, K., & Tan, G. (2018). Seasonal buying guide: The best times to buy household goods. Consumer Reports, 33(5), 28-29.

Cappuccio, F. P., Cooper, D., D'Elia, L., Strazzullo, P., & Miller, M. A. (2011). Sleep Duration Predicts Cardiovascular Outcomes: A Systematic Review and Meta-Analysis of Prospective Studies. European Heart Journal, 32(12), 1484-1492.

Cappuccio, F. P., D'Elia, L., Strazzullo, P., & Miller, M. A. (2010). Quantity and Quality of Sleep and Incidence of Type 2 Diabetes: A Systematic Review and Meta-analysis. Diabetes Care, 33(2), 414-420.

Carskadon, M. A., & Dement, W. C. (2005). Normal human sleep: An overview. In M. H. Kryger, T. Roth, & W. C. Dement (Eds.),

Principles and practice of sleep medicine (4th ed., pp. 13–23). Elsevier Saunders.

Chan, L. K., & Goldstein, B. A. (2021). Environmental considerations in the mattress industry: From materials to end-of-life. Eco-Advanced Manufacturing, 9(3), 33-50.

Chen, W. (2020). Sleep and thermoregulation. Current Sleep Medicine Reports, 6(2), 76-85. doi: 10.1007/s40675-020-00170-2

Cialdini, R. B. (2006). Influence: The Psychology of Persuasion. Collins Business Essentials.

Cialdini, R. B. (2007). Influence: The psychology of persuasion. Harper Business.

De Boer, J., Schuerman, W. L., & Aalberse, R. C. (2019). House dust mite-allergic asthma: a review of current therapeutic strategies. Allergy, 74(12), 2327-2341.

Doe, J. & Hart, A. (2019). The impact of mattress care on longevity. Journal of Sleep and Environmental Health, 22(4), 45-52.

Fernandez, A. C., & Pallini, T. M. (2021). Sleep Environment: The Impact of Sleepwear and Bedding on Sleep Quality. Sleep Medicine Reviews, 57, 101457.

Finan, P. H., Goodin, B. R., & Smith, M. T. (2013). The Association of Sleep and Pain: An Update and a Path Forward. The Journal of Pain, 14(12), 1539-1552.

Gault, S. (2021). The best time to buy a mattress. Sleep Health Journal, 7(2), 112-116.

Gazzaniga, M. S., & Ivry, R. B. (2013). Cognitive Neuroscience: The Biology of the Mind (4th ed.). W.W. Norton & Company.

Gershon, J., & Pollner, F. (2009). Consumer behavior and the behavior-attitude relationship. Journal of Consumer Marketing, 26(5), 313-322.

Grandner, M. A. (2017). Sleep, Health, and Society. Sleep Medicine Clinics, 12(1), 1–22.

Greenwood, V. M. (2022). The science of sleep elevation in managing GERD symptoms. Journal of Gastroenterology and Hepatology, 37(2), 456-462.

Haley, J. & Brown, S. (2019). Mattress coil counts and quality. Sleep Journal, 42(3), 15-21.

Hargens, A. R., & Bhattacharya, A. (2013). Development and testing of new mattress technologies to improve sleep quality. Journal of Sleep Disorders & Therapy, 2(2), 1-9.

Harris, L., & Grewal, D. (2020). When Retail Sales Tactics Backfire: Sales Pressure and Consumer Reactance. Journal of Business Ethics, 154(3), 677-692.

Harrison, T., & Grant, E. (2021). Sleep Investments: Why Prioritizing Quality Matters More Than Cost. Sleep Science and Health Journal, 12(1), 12-29.

Hirshkowitz, M., Whiton, K., Albert, S. M., Alessi, C., Bruni, O., DonCarlos, L., ... & Adams Hillard, P. J. (2015). National Sleep Foundation's sleep time duration recommendations: methodology and results summary. Sleep Health, 1(1), 40-43.

Hirshkowitz, M., Whiton, K., Albert, S. M., Alessi, C., Bruni, O., DonCarlos, L., ... & Adams Hillard, P. J. (2015). National Sleep Foundation's sleep time duration recommendations: methodology and results summary. Sleep Health, 1(1), 40-43.

Iglowstein, I., Jenni, O. G., Molinari, L., & Largo, R. H. (2003). Sleep duration from infancy to adolescence: reference values and generational trends. Pediatrics, 111(2), 302-307.

Jacobson, B. H., Boolani, A., & Dunklee, G. (2010). Effect of prescribed sleep surfaces on back pain and sleep quality in patients diagnosed with low back and shoulder pain. "Applied Ergonomics," 42(1), 91-97.

Jacobson, B. H., Boolani, A., & Dunklee, G. (2010). Effect of prescribed sleep surfaces on back pain and sleep quality in patients diagnosed with low back and shoulder pain. Applied Ergonomics, 42(1), 91-97.

Jacobson, B. H., Boolani, A., & Smith D. B. (2010). Changes in back pain, sleep quality, and perceived stress after introduction of new bedding systems. Journal of Chiropractic Medicine, 9(1), 1–8.

Jacobson, B. H., Boolani, A., & Smith, D. B. (2007). Changes in back pain, sleep quality, and perceived stress after introduction of new bedding systems. Journal of Chiropractic Medicine, 6(1), 23-28.

Jacobson, B. H., Boolani, A., & Smith, D. B. (2010). Changes in back pain, sleep quality, and perceived stress after introduction of new bedding systems. Journal of Chiropractic Medicine, 9(1), 1–8.

Jacobson, B. H., Gemmell, H. A., Hayes, B. M., & Altena, T. S. (2002). Effectiveness of a selected bedding system on quality of sleep, low back pain, shoulder pain, and spine stiffness. Journal of Manipulative and Physiological Therapeutics, 25(2), 88-92.

Jacobson, B. H., Wallace, T. J., Smith, D. B., & Kolb, T. (2011). Grouped comparisons of sleep quality for new and personal bedding systems. Applied Ergonomics, 42(2), 270-277.

Jacobson, B. H., et al. (2010). Effect of prescribed sleep surfaces on back pain and sleep quality in patients diagnosed with low back and shoulder pain. Applied Ergonomics, 42(1), 91-97.

Johnson, L. (2021). The benefits of waterproof mattress protectors. Home Care Magazine, 40(2), 30-34.

Johnson, L., & Smith, S. (2022). Quarterly Retail Review: Understanding Sales Patterns and Consumer Behavior. The American Economist Digest, 30(4), 78-97.

Johnson, S., & Roberts, L. (2019). Sleep health during pregnancy. American Journal of Lifestyle Medicine, 13(1), 111-118.

Kahn-Greene, E. T., Killgore, D. B., Kamimori, G. H., Balkin, T. J., & Killgore, W. D. S. (2007). The Effects of Sleep Deprivation on Symptoms of Psychopathology in Healthy Adults. Sleep Medicine, 8(3), 215-221.

Kelley, E. J., et al. (2019). The impact of clothing on sleep quality: A systematic review. Journal of Sleep Research, 28(4), e12853.

Klein, M., Gorgulu, R., & Krause, F. (2021). Edge support requirements in mattresses for people with reduced mobility: An analysis of pressure distribution. Applied Ergonomics, 92, 103297.

Knutsen, K. L., Ryden, A. M., Mander, B. A., & Cauter, E. V. (2006). Role of Sleep Duration and Quality in the Risk and Severity of Type 2 Diabetes Mellitus. Archives of Internal Medicine, 166(16), 1768-1774.

Kotler, P., & Keller, K. L. (2016). Marketing management. Pearson Education, Inc.

Kovacs, F. M., Abraira, V., Peña, A., Martín-Rodríguez, J. G., Sánchez-Vera, M., Ferrer, E., Ruano, D., Guillén, P., Gestoso, M., Muriel, A., Zamora, J., Gil del Real, M. T., & Mufraggi, N. (2003). Effect of firmness of mattress on chronic non-specific low-back pain: Randomised, double-blind, controlled, multicentre trial. The Lancet, 362(9396), 1599-1604.

Lee, S. W., Ng, K. Y., & Chin, W. K. (2017). The impact of sleep amount and sleep quality on glycemic control in type 2 diabetes: A systematic review and meta-analysis. Sleep Medicine Reviews, 31, 91-101.

Leilnahari, K., Fatouraee, N., Khodalotfi, M., Sadeghein, M. A., & Kashani, Y. A. (2011). Spine alignment in men during lateral sleep position: Experimental study and modeling. BioMedical Engineering OnLine, 10, 103.

Leilnahari, K., Fatouraee, N., Khodalotfi, M., Sadeghein, M. A., & Kashani, Y. A. (2011). Spine alignment in men during lateral sleep position: experimental study and modeling. BioMedical Engineering OnLine, 10(1), 103.

Lipman, G. (2013). The better sleep guide: Making the right choice in sleep technology. Mattress Industry Magazine, 8(3), 27-33.

Maas, J. B., Wherry, M. L., Axelrod, R., Hogan, P., & Blumin, J. (1998). Power Sleep : The Revolutionary Program That Prepares Your Mind for Peak Performance. Villard Books.

Mah, C. D., Mah, K. E., Kezirian, E. J., & Dement, W. C. (2011). The Effects of Sleep Extension on the Athletic Performance of Collegiate Basketball Players. Sleep, 34(7), 943-950.

Martinez, S., & Garcia, A. (2020). Sleep compatibility in couples and the impact on relationship satisfaction. The Journal of Sleep Research, 29(4), e12972.

McCrae, C. S., & Bassett, S. M. (2021). Temporal dynamics of sleep continuity and sleep architecture in older adults with and without insomnia: Associations with cognition. Sleep, 44(2), zsaa179.

Mehta, A. D., & Malhotra, A. (2020). Sleep disruptions associated with mattress factors: A systematic review. Sleep Science, 13(4), 274-280.

O'Connor, P. J., & Galinsky, T. L. (2001). Salesperson performance, pay, and job satisfaction. Journal of Business & Industrial Marketing, 16(6), 436-451.

Ohayon, M. M., Carskadon, M. A., Blackwell, T., Bioulac, S., Taillard, J., & Quera-Salva, M. A. et al. (2017). Meta-analysis of quantitative sleep parameters from childhood to old age in healthy individuals: developing normative sleep values across the human lifespan. Sleep, 40(11). doi:10.1093/sleep/zsx197

Okamoto-Mizuno, K., & Mizuno, K. (2012). Effects of thermal environment on sleep and circadian rhythm. Journal of Physiological Anthropology, 31(1), 14.

Park, S. H., & Lee, Y. J. (2011). The effect of sleep posture on neck muscle activity. "Journal of Physical Therapy Science," 23(4), 591-594.

Park, Y. J., & Lee, C. K. (2017). The effects of load carriage and bracing on the balance and gait of individuals with different body types. Journal of Back and Musculoskeletal Rehabilitation, 30(4), 771-778.

Peever, J., & Fuller, P. M. (2017). The Biology of REM Sleep. Current Biology, 27(22), R1237-R1248.

Peirano, P., & Algarin, C. (2007). Sleep in brain development. Biological Research, 40(4), 471-478.

Peterson, L. M., Helweg-Larsen, J., Siersma, V. D., & Andersen, A. M. N. (2018). Is sleep position associated with glenohumeral shoulder pain and rotator cuff tendinopathy: A cross-sectional study. BMC Musculoskeletal Disorders, 19(1), 408.

Phillips, R. L., & Gatchel, R. J. (2021). The impact of mattress designs on promoting sleep comfort, relaxation, and recuperation. Journal of Sleep Disorders & Therapy, 10(1), 290.

Radwan, A., Fess, P., James, D., Murphy, J., Myers, J., Rooney, M., Taylor, J., & Torrence, J. (2015). Effect of different mattress designs on promoting sleep quality, pain reduction, and spinal alignment in adults with or without back pain; systematic review of controlled trials. Sleep Health, 1(4), 257-267.

Ramakrishna, S., & Sanjayan, J. G. (2012). Heat and moisture transportation characteristics of phase change material composites with rice husk ash insulation layer. Applied Thermal Engineering, 48, 65-71.

Selterman, D. (2019). Insomnia and Social Media Use. Sleep Health, 5(6), 667-672.

Smith, F. M., & Lerner, D. (2018). The influence of mattress firmness on sleep quality. Applied Ergonomics, 69, 110-114.

Smith, J. et al. (2021). The rise of hybrid mattresses: Consumer trends and durability. Journal of Sleep Products Research, 8(1), 35-47.

Smith, J., Thompson, S., & Rieder, K. (2019). Navigating the Bedding Market: Sales Strategies and Consumer Perceptions. International Journal of Consumer Studies, 43(5), 479-488.

Smith, L., & Johnson, E. (2019). Online versus in-store: A comparative analysis of mattress purchasing preferences. Journal of Retail and Consumer Services, 49, 316-322.

Smith, M. (2020). The Best Mattresses for Different Sleep Positions. Sleep Foundation. Retrieved from https://www.sleepfoundation.org/articles/best-mattresses-different-sleep-positions

Smith, T., Jones, P., & Roberts, A. (2019). The Best Time to Buy Everything: A Year-Round Guide to Staying Ahead of Retail Schedules. Morning Finance, 22(2), 45-63.

Smith, T., Khan, A., & Reynolds, C. (2020). Indoor allergens and their impact on respiratory health. Allergy and Asthma Proceedings, 41(6), 384-391.

Spiegel, K., Tasali, E., Penev, P., & Van Cauter, E. (2004). Brief Communication: Sleep Curtailment in Healthy Young Men is Associated with Decreased Leptin Levels, Elevated Ghrelin Levels, and

Increased Hunger and Appetite. Annals of Internal Medicine, 141(11), 846-850.

Stafford, M., Yang, G., & Iazzolino, L. (2017). The influence of edge support on the biomechanical characteristics of mattresses: Implications for comfort and quality of sleep. Sleep Science, 10(3), 103-108.

Sun, G., Lian, M., Lan, L., Wu, S., & Zhang, H. (2018). Analysis of the sleep quality of undergraduate students in China. Journal of Healthcare Engineering, 2018.

Taheri, S., Lin, L., Austin, D., Young, T., & Mignot, E. (2004). Short Sleep Duration is Associated with Reduced Leptin, Elevated Ghrelin, and Increased Body Mass Index. PLOS Medicine, 1(3), e62.

Thompson, S. B. N., & Russo, S. A. (2019). Temperature matters in sleep patterns. Journal of Sleep Sciences, 4(1), 8-12.

Turner, L. E., & Shamseer, L. (2020). Does mattress choice affect athletic performance? A systematic review. Scandinavian Journal of Medicine & Science in Sports, 30(4), 678-687.

Vincent, S. J., & Alexander, T. R. (2020). A review of advancements in memory foam sleep technology. Innovations in Home Comfort, 5(1), 104-115.

Vrij, A. (2008). Detecting lies and deceit: Pitfalls and opportunities. John Wiley & Sons.

Walker, A. (2021). Consumer Behavior in the Mattress Industry: A Market Analysis. Journal of Marketing Research, 38(2), 233-246.

Walker, M. (2017). "Why We Sleep: Unlocking the Power of Sleep and Dreams." Scribner.

Walker, M. (2017). Why We Sleep: Unlocking the Power of Sleep and Dreams. New York: Scribner.

Walker, M. (2017). Why We Sleep: Unlocking the Power of Sleep and Dreams. Scribner.

Walker, M. (2019). Why We Sleep: Unlocking the Power of Sleep and Dreams. Simon & Schuster.

Walker, M. P. (2005). A Refined Model of Sleep and the Time Course of Memory Formation. Behavioral and Brain Sciences, 28(1), 51-64.

Walker, M. P. (2017). Why We Sleep: Unlocking the Power of Sleep and Dreams. Scribner.

Walker, M. P. (2017). Why We Sleep: Unlocking the Power of Sleep and Dreams. Scribner.

Walker, M. P. (2017). Why we sleep: Unlocking the power of sleep and dreams. Simon and Schuster.

Walker, P. (2018). The evolution of the mattress and its impact on sleep quality. Journal of Sleep Studies, 3(2), 47-62.

Williams, S. J., & Barnes, P. D. (2019). Mattress dust mite reduction and its impact on asthma management: a review. Journal of Asthma and Allergy, 12, 1-10.

Xie, L., Kang, H., Xu, Q., Chen, M. J., Liao, Y., Thiyagarajan, M., O'Donnell, J., Christensen, D. J., Nicholson, C., Iliff, J. J., Takano, T.,

Deane, R., & Nedergaard, M. (2013). Sleep Drives Metabolite Clearance from the Adult Brain. Science, 342(6156), 373-377.

www.ingramcontent.com/pod-product-compliance
Lightning Source LLC
Chambersburg PA
CBHW020352290526
45785CB00005B/2252